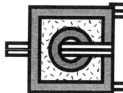 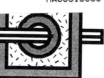

Leisure Step Up Workbook

Welcome to our program and the **Leisure Step Up Workbook**. Participation will help you learn positive directions for solving problems, meeting needs **and** leading a healthy leisure lifestyle.

by Dave Dehn, CTRS, CLP

Idyll Arbor, Inc.

PO Box 720, Ravensdale, WA 98051 (425) 432-3231

Published and Distributed by

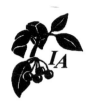

Idyll Arbor, Inc.

PO Box 720, Ravensdale, WA 98051 (425) 432-3231

ISBN 1-882883-18-7

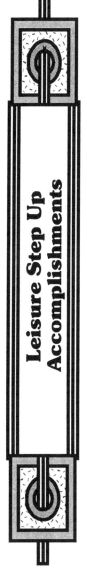

Leisure Step Up Accomplishments

Step Number	Description of Step	Date Accomplished	Staff Initial	Participant Initial	Comments
Step 1	Step Up Leisure Assessment				
Step 2	Leisure Problem Descriptions				
Step 3	Leisure Education Part ☐ A, ☐ B, ☐ C, ☐ D, ☐ E, ☐ F				
Step 4	Recreation Participation				
Step 5	Leisure of the Past				
Step 6	Leisure of the Future				
Step 7	Community Spectator Participation				
Step 8	Expressive Leisure Participation				
Step 9	Physical Leisure Participation				
Step 10	Cultural Leisure Participation				
Step 11	Post - Discharge Recreation Participation				

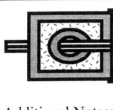

Leisure Step Up
Accomplishments

Additional Notes:

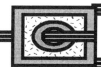

Step 1
Leisure Assessment

Directions: Please read each question carefully, being honest with each question. After you read each sentence, indicate how much that sentence describes how you feel using the scale below.

1. Almost Never	2. Rarely	3. Sometimes	4. Usually	5. Almost Always

Leisure Functioning

____ 1. The things I do with my free time are positive.

____ 2. I get to do the things I want to with my free time.

____ 3. I enjoy my free time.

____ 4. When I get free time, I do not know what to do.

____ 5. I get enough free time.

____ 6. I am interested in learning new things to do.

____ 7. My free time is boring.

Physical Functioning

____ 1. I like the way I look.

____ 2. I am physically active.

____ 3. I feel good physically.

____ 4. My physical health and condition prevent me from doing what I want.

____ 5. I get enough sleep.

____ 6. I have enough energy.

____ 7. My drug or alcohol use creates problems.

Cognitive Functioning

____ 1. I can concentrate or focus on a task.

____ 2. I can participate in the same activity for a long period of time.

____ 3. I can think clearly in solving my problems.

____ 4. I forget things that happened to me and what I did when I was young.

____ 5. I know where I am, what day it is and what I am doing.

____ 6. I understand directions or rules.

____ 7. Ten minutes after I see, read or hear something I forget what it was.

Daily Living Functioning

____ 1. I feel safe in my home.

____ 2. I eat a balanced diet.

____ 3. I bathe or shower daily and take care of my health.

____ 4. I have problems with those I work or go to school with.

____ 5. I attend my school or job.

____ 6. I participate in cleaning, cooking and responsibilities at home.

____ 7. I have problems with school/job or my daily responsibilities.

Social Functioning

____ 1. I share my feelings.

____ 2. I can depend upon my friends.

____ 3. I get along with authority.

____ 4. I avoid time alone.

____ 5. My family is important to me.

____ 6. I enjoy being around others.

____ 7. I give in to peer pressure.

Psychological Functioning

____ 1. I think positively about myself.

____ 2. My stress level is manageable.

____ 3. I make good decisions.

____ 4. I feel depressed.

____ 5. I am calm and in control.

____ 6. I behave in a rational manner.

____ 7. My attitude leads to problems.

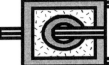

Step 1
Assessment Summary

Functional Ability:

Leisure Functioning: _____

Physical Functioning: _____

Cognitive Functioning: _____

Daily Living Functioning: _____

Social Functioning: _____

Psychological Functioning: _____

Global Assessment and Leisure Functioning (GALF) SCALE: _____

Comments/Summary:

Treatment Goals and Objectives:

Participant _____ Date _____ Staff _____
© Copyright 1995 Dehn and Idyll Arbor, Inc.

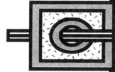

Step 1
Information Handout

Name _____ **Date** _____

Directions: Please fill in the blank spaces provided.

My main reason for coming in for treatment is _____

_____

_____

Things I do with my free time include:

_____   _____

_____   _____

Things that prevent me from doing what I want are

_____   _____

_____   _____

List any physical/health problems or allergies:

_____   _____

_____   _____

I am employed or have been employed in the past: ☐ No ☐ Yes

If Yes, ☐ Past ☐ Currently

My job was/is _____ I work(ed) _____ hours per week

If I had any problems with my job, it was _____

_____

I currently attend school: ☐ No ☐ Yes

If Yes, I am in the _____ grade.

My average grades are _____.

My relationships with teachers are

☐ pleasant   ☐ friendly   ☐ so-so   ☐ unfriendly   ☐ disgusting

Explain: _____

_____

My relationships with peers are _____

_____

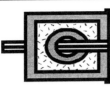

Step 1
Information Handout

Additional Information:

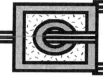 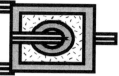

Step 2 Part A
Problem Descriptions

Name _____   **Date** _____

Directions: List three major problems and write a brief description of each problem.

1. Problem:

   Description:

2. Problem:

   Description:

3. Problem:

   Description:

4. Other problem areas include:

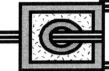
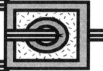

Step 2 Part B
Problem Solutions

Name _____ Date _____

Directions: With the help of the recreational therapist, write down recreation and leisure goals which will help solve the problems you listed.

1. Problem:

    Leisure Goal:

2. Problem:

    Leisure Goal:

3. Problem:

    Leisure Goal:

4. Other goals include:

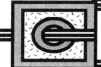 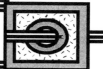

Step 3 Checklist

Name _____   **Date** _____

Directions: Use this checklist to keep track of the parts of Step 3.

A) The Leisure Level Model. Part A will tell you about positive and negative leisure behaviors.

   Completed _____

B) Leisure Participation Level. Part B will give you information about your leisure participation level.

   Completed _____

C) Leisure Attitude Awareness Stems. Part C will help you understand your attitude toward leisure activities.

   Completed _____

D) Days In My Life. Part D will identify your use of time during a typical 24 hour day.

   Completed _____

E) Leisure Resources. Part E will tell you about basic home and community leisure resources.

   Completed _____

F) Things I Enjoy. Part F will identify your leisure interests and areas of enjoyment.

   Completed _____

Leisure Level Model

The activities that I choose to participate in during my free time.

Healthy Positive Choices ⇑ ⇑

Unhealthy Negative Choices ⇓ ⇓

Cathartic Level

My Choices/My Behavior. My participation reaches a point of catharsis. My participation makes a measurable change in my life. **Examples:** vacation, climbing a mountain, prayer, ropes course, watching an event, achieving the goal, etc.

Level 4

My Choices/My Behavior. I am creative, inventive, imaginative, taking nothing and making something. Not following a plan or instruction. **Examples:** Poetry, drawing, painting, crafts, cooking, sculpting, music, prayer, etc.

Level 3

My Choices/My Behavior. I am active physically, socially and/or cognitively. Activity follows instruction, a plan, rules, with participation on an emotional level. **Examples:** Crafts, cooking, bike riding, sports participation, intense laughter (internal jogging), dancing, games, skateboarding, reading, physical workout, relaxation therapy, etc.

Level 2

My Choices/My Behavior. I am a spectator emotionally involved. There is a personal investment, true entertainment. **Examples:** TV, radio, watching others participate in Level 3 and 4 activities.

Level 1

My Choices/My Behavior. I am a spectator with no emotional involvement. Participation lacks personal investment, *positive* activities with nothing else to do. **Examples:** Watching TV, listening to the radio, watching others participate in Level 3 and 4 activities.

Level 0

My Choices/My Behavior. I am preoccupied in thought or feeling and just going through the motions of the activity. Participation could be forced, obligated, duty, with no internalization of participation. **Examples:**
Preoccupation during participation in Level 1, 2, 3 or 4 activities.

Level -1

My Choices/My Behavior. I am harmed physically, mentally or emotionally. **Examples:** Substance abuse, dangerous high risk activities, self abuse, negative thinking, poor dietary choices, too much or not enough sleeping, eating, exercising, relaxing, etc.

Level -2

My Choices/My Behavior. I affect others in a harmful or hurting manner. This includes physical, emotional or mental harm to my family, friends or community. **Examples:** Substance abuse, inappropriate competition, gossip, threatening, name calling, fighting, hurting animals, breaking the law (minor), no family time, etc.

Lost Freedom

My Choices/My Behavior. I harm myself or others. My behavior causes a loss in freedom to choose my own leisure. Often the victim's and/or family's leisure are also affected. **Examples:** Crime, gang involvement, vandalism, fighting, suicide gestures, breaking the law (major: rape, self abuse, sexual abuse, substance abuse, etc.).

Explanation of the Leisure Levels

Level 0: Preoccupied

Level 0 is neither a positive or a negative level. It is when you are pre-occupied in thought or feeling and will get little to no benefits from participating in an upper level activity.

When your thoughts or feelings are not connected with what you are doing, you are not really "into" the activity. You are there physically, but nothing else. Pre-occupation many times is on work, problem areas, responsibilities, things you think you really should be doing, feelings of guilt, depression, anger, frustration, etc.

An example that you might identify with: Suppose you go on a weekend vacation (to a fantastic place) but the whole time you are there you are pre-occupied about a poor relationship, fear of what could happen during the weekend, worrying about past abuse issues, etc. You might as well have stayed home, since you are functioning on Level 0 and are not really mentally and emotionally at this fantastic place.

You may also be participating at Level 0 when you are forced to do something by outside pressure or influence. An example of this: you feel obligated to attend a family function that you do not wish to attend. It may be a duty or you may feel forced. Because of this pressure you may not internalize the participation, thus you are participating at Level 0.

An exception to this would be if you are pre-occupied with a problem area, solving or partially solving the problem during leisure participation. Problem solving during leisure is participation on a therapeutic level. For example, if you take the weekend vacation to a fantastic place and it solves or deals with a problem about a poor relationship, fear of the unknown, past abuse issues, etc., then you are participating on a therapeutic level which is extremely positive and healthy. Other examples include: 1) engaging in physical activity or exercise when you are pre-occupied with anger, hurt, frustration, etc. and you release feelings through participation; 2) engaging in poetry, story writing, journalizing, art, crafts, music, etc. to express or deal with problem areas; 3) watching a movie, reading a book, listening to a song, etc., vicariously solving your problems through emotional involvement as a spectator.

The therapeutic level is the outcome of the Leisure Plan from Step 2. It is the difference between leisure participation in drama and therapeutic participation in psychodrama. The difference between social talking in a group and a group therapy session. The difference between talking with someone and a therapeutic individual session. The difference between a family talking and a therapeutic family session. It is truly getting your needs met by solving problems.

Level -1: Harm To Myself

Level -1 is the first level in the unhealthy negative direction. It is when your participation during leisure is harmful to yourself. There may not be an initial problem created by participation, but if you continue, you will eventually be less healthy. Examples of this include smoking cigarettes, eating junk food, lack of activity, etc. Another example, would be when you participate in an activity such as bowling, skiing, crafts, etc. with negative thoughts such as: I'm dumb, I'll never learn how to do this, I always look stupid trying something new, I must be the dumbest person here, etc.

A key factor in this level is too much or not enough. Often times it is difficult to determine how much is too much or how little is too little. A good rule of thumb is, if doing something causes you trouble — even a little bit, it is probably a Level -1 activity. Some examples might be watching a violent movie, reading an over stimulating sex book, listening to negative messages in music, etc. Often participation in these activities lead to Level -2 or Lost Freedom.

Keep in mind that you need to be very careful not to say something is okay for you when it really isn't. Your therapist and others around you may be seeing it more clearly than you are.

Level -2: Harm To Others

Level -2 is the second level of unhealthy negative choices. At times your participation on Level -1 will fall to Level -2 as the ways you are hurting yourself start to hurt others. Examples include: addictions to drugs, alcohol, gambling, sex or work which harms members of your family. A good test for whether you are harming others is not what you think, but how others tell you they feel. It's hard to admit to yourself that you are hurting the ones you love, but if they say it is so, you should at least admit that it might be true.

You might consider participation on this level as fun, exciting or a means of self expression. This can be true, but if your actions also hurt others, they are unhealthy and negative. Sooner or later they will bring harm and hurt to you or others. Having fun at someone else's expense is also a poor choice in leisure. Examples include: ethnic jokes, stealing, destruction of property, gossip and lying about an individual. These are all Level -2 activities.

Lost Freedom

Lost Freedom cannot be given a negative number, as even participation in positive levels cannot balance your leisure life. Participation on this level has a drastic effect upon you and others affected by your behavior. It is extremely important for you to have a clear understanding of this level if you have experienced this level first hand, either as a participant or as a victim.

If you participate on this level, you may lose your freedom by having to deal with consequences such as negative self feelings, thoughts and self esteem. You are not locked into this level and through therapeutic intervention you may change your leisure lifestyle and deal with issues causing your behaviors. Examples include: harm from drunk driving, rape, serious injury due to fighting, going to prison for stealing, etc.

If you have been a victim of a violent action, you may also be on this level, especially if you experience extreme feelings of fear, guilt, anger, along with thoughts of low self esteem, lack of interest or vindictiveness. Being a victim of violence has a tremendous effect on your freedom in choosing leisure. Therapeutic intervention may restore your positive thoughts and feelings, enabling you to choose of a healthy leisure lifestyle.

You are also participating at this level if you are pre-occupied with suicidal thoughts, involved in self abuse or suicidal gestures. Violent acts against yourself cloud your mind and decision making ability, limiting your freedom to make healthy/positive leisure choices. Examples: cutting oneself with a razor blade, suicide attempts, pre-occupation with extreme negative and suicidal thought, gang fighting with no self concern, sexual promiscuity with no protection, etc. Therapeutic intervention is helpful and many times necessary to help you regain a healthy leisure lifestyle.

Level 1: Uninvolved Spectator

Level 1 participation is on the low end of positive healthy participation. When you first look at this level, it may appear of little value. There are, however, times when your mind, body and emotions are fatigued and you need to do nothing. Our culture has stringent demands for both work and play and it can be hard for you to do nothing (and not feel guilty). You are on this level if you are a spectator with no emotional investment. Examples are watching cars drive by while sitting on the porch, resting while listening to background music, attending a sporting event with no concern for outcome, etc.

Level 2: Involved Spectator

Level 2 is similar to Level 1, except that you are emotionally involved as a spectator. You are on this level when you are interested and experiencing or expressing an emotion. Examples are going to a sad movie, reading a dramatic book, watching a love story on TV, attending an emotionally charged basketball game, attending a museum with a high interest in the art work, etc. You must be careful in this area, as we live in a society that wants to be entertained. TV, for example, monopolizes many lives. If you spend all of your time watching TV (or playing Nintendo), you are on Level -1 not Level 2. Too much TV or Nintendo is just not good for you.

Level 3: Active Participation

Level 3 participation is an upper level in the Leisure Level Model continuum. When defining recreation most people think of activity on this level. If you are on this level you are a player, a participant as opposed to a spectator as in Levels 1 and 2. It includes cognitive, physical and social parts. You need to think. You need to move your body. You need to interact with others. And you need to be able to perform tasks requiring significant levels of coordination. One is not a substitute for the other, as we must participate in some element of physical, social and cognitive activity on a regular basic to be healthy. A key point in this level is following a plan, instruction or rules during participation.

The physical category is extremely important in therapy and needs to be a part of all of our lives in maintaining health. Physical activity and exercise may be the most used and highly accepted therapeutic programming approach in recreational therapy. If you have been inactive or if you are in poor physical condition, you must be careful when you start to do more physical exercise. Talk with your doctor before you begin an exercise program. Examples of physical participation include: riding a bike, fly fishing, weight training, walking a nature trail, following an instructor in aerobic exercise, playing racquetball, jogging or dancing the fox-trot.

The cognitive category includes the thinking process. Your participation in cognitive aspects are important because thinking clearly is important in solving problems. Participation in cognitive activities sharpens our thought process leading to improved decision making, listening skills, improved memory, etc. Examples of cognitive participation are reading a "how to repair" book, playing a game of strategy, chess, Clue, Memory, reminiscing while watching home movies, working on puzzles, math problems, word problems or following instructions in building a model ship.

The social category includes verbal and/or non-verbal conversation/interaction with at least one other person. Your participation must include emotional involvement or the socialization would be on a lower level. You may think sitting down with a friend and carrying on a conversation or being at a party or engagement with a group as the only way to be social. Socialization also includes non-verbal participation in recreation activities. The action, the play, the movement are your means of communication. Examples include playing checkers, basketball, table games, sport activity and group projects.

It is not necessarily important to decide if an activity is physical, social or cognitive. The decision however would be which aspects are considered important during participation.

For a healthy leisure you need to have some of each. How you mix and match your activities to get them all is ultimately up to you.

Level 4: Creative Participation

Level 4 participation offers a means of expressing your emotions. It is above Level 3 in emotive expression, in that your participation does not follow a plan, pattern or instruction. You leave part of yourself in what you accomplish and what you accomplish becomes part of you. Many poets, artists and musicians describe this level of participation as including their soul, the essence of their existence. A key phrase is taking nothing and making something. Examples are taking a lump of clay and molding a figure, writing a short story, cooking from scratch (no recipe), talking to God from your heart, making plans to decorate for a party or unstructured free play.

Contrary to what you may believe, this level can be achieved by learning and practicing. Some people say, "I'm not a creative person." However, creativity can be learned. Just like all good things, it takes work (or play, depending on your perception of leisure) to be successfully creative.

Cathartic Level: Growth Through Participation

Cathartic Level is the ultimate level in leisure participation. It is free time participation that is extremely emotional. When you are participating in Level 2, 3 or 4 activities, you may reach a cathartic point. It is your personal growth that many times acts as a catalyst for a change in your lifestyle. Many times you cannot plan to achieve this level. It happens as a result of the right chemistry of your emotional state and the activity. It is participation on a Level 2, 3 or 4 that has a lasting and memorable effect on you. Examples are watching a movie that portrays an aspect of your life teaching you new values, talking to God and gaining inspiration, going on a family vacation that solidifies family ties.

Summary

The Leisure Level Model is a tool that gives value to choices and behaviors during leisure time. It can help you see that what you do with your leisure time does make a difference and it gives you a goal to achieve. You do not always need to participate on a high level. You need to find a balance among the positive Levels 1 through 4, while staying away from participation on the negative levels.

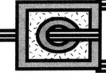

Step 3 Part B
Leisure Participation

Name _____   Date _____

A. Leisure Activities that I have participated in within the last 30 days	B. Leisure Level		C. Times I participated in the last 30 days		D. Activity Points
		X		=	
		X		=	
		X		=	
		X		=	
		X		=	
		X		=	
		X		=	
		X		=	
		X		=	
		X		=	
		X		=	
		X		=	
		X		=	
		X		=	
		X		=	
		X		=	
		X		=	
		X		=	
		X		=	
Totals for columns C and D					

Level of Participation: Total of Column D divided by Total of Column C _____

My thoughts about my level of participation ...

My feelings about how I spend my time are ...

A) List the leisure or recreational activities that you have participated in within the last 30 days, including positive and negative activities. List at least 10 activities.

B) Give each activity points from the Leisure Level Model.

C) Fill in how many times you have participated in each activity within the last 30 days.

D) Multiply column B times column C and put the answer in column D.

E) Count up the number of times you participated in activities in column C and put it at the bottom of column C.

F) Add or subtract in column D to get the total and put it at the bottom of column D.

G) Divide the total in column D by the total number of activities in column C to get your average level of participation shown in the chart below.

Leisure Participation Scale

Cathartic Level	Participation in at least one leisure activity with a great deal of emotional release. The event resulted in personal growth.
Level 4	Participation is creative, inventive, imaginative. Be cautious to not spend excessive time in your own world.
Level 2 to 4	Participation seems to be in balance. Leisure pursuits are enjoyable, expressive, active and helpful in solving problems.
Level 1 to 2	Participation spectator. Be cautious that you don't let life pass you by. Also, negative/harmful activity participation can jeopardize the balance in your life.
Level 0	Participation co-dependent. You need to talk, trust, feel, think and live for yourself. Perhaps unhealthy, negative choices are highly influencing your behaviors.
Level -1 to -2	Participation harmful/hurting. These choices may seem fun and harmless but are often driven by anger or unmet needs. Leisure counseling and education can help you attain a higher leisure level or quality of life.
Lost Freedom	Counseling may be necessary to restoring you to a healthy, positive level of participation. Seek help, direction and support from a friend, family member, clergy or counselor. Freedom can be restored and it is worth the trouble.

Note: Quality of leisure is not just how many points you scored. Participation at a high level alone does not necessarily mean that you are enjoying yourself. Also you must not get discouraged with a low score. Since you control your own leisure choices, you can change toward healthy positive choices.

Step 3 Part C
Leisure Attitude Awareness

Name _____   Date _____

Please complete each stem and write a brief explanation

1) Most important at a party or social engagement is ...

2) When I have time alone, I feel ...

3) When I think of physical activity and exercise, I ...

4) My free time at home is ...

5) I express myself best in recreation activities that I ...

6) I believe my leisure time would be more positive if ...

7) When I was younger, my attitude toward free time was ...

8) I like to keep in shape physically by ...

9) I believe what I do during my free time affects my self esteem because ...

10) When there is work needing to be done and I have free time, I think ...

11) My attitude toward my family doing leisure activities and spending time together is ...

12) I believe my accomplishments at work or school are enhanced by my leisure activities because ...

13) When I think of activities, where I have to use my brain I ...

My Thoughts —

My Feelings —

My Ideas —

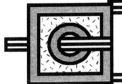
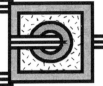

Step 3 Part D
Days In My Life

Name _____   Date _____

Fill in <u>specifically</u> how you spend your time in a typical 24 hour day.

Days In My Life	Weekday	Weekend
7:00 am		
8:00 am		
9:00 am		
10:00 am		
11:00 am		
12:00 pm		
1:00 pm		
2:00 pm		
3:00 pm		
4:00 pm		
5:00 pm		
6:00 pm		
7:00 pm		
8:00 pm		
9:00 pm		
10:00 pm		
11:00 pm		
12:00 am		
1:00 am		
2:00 am		
3:00 am		
4:00 am		
5:00 am		
6:00 am		

Step 3 Part D
Days In My Life

My thoughts about:

1) The amount of time I spend with my family ...

2) The amount of sleep I get ...

3) The amount of time I participate in healthy leisure activities ...

4) The most positive thing I do with my time is ...

5) I would like to change ...

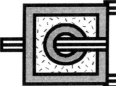

Step 3 Part E
Crossword Puzzle

Community Resources — DOWN

A) This city resource has pamphlets and information of community events _____ of Commerce.

B) This activity requires a cold floor and funny shoes — 2 words.

C) This activity used to be called nine pins.

D) A place to go to learn of the past or the future and see important items, pictures and stories.

E) Here, I can study animals and observe them as they are in the wild.

F) This sport is getting more and more popular, probably due to the challenge, the beauty of the course and the walk that includes 18 holes.

G) If I did not get my high school diploma, I can attend classes and study to get these initials.

H) Depending upon the weather, I may go barefoot, need boots or wear comfortable shoes to participate in this aerobic activity. I could go with my neighbor or take my dog when I go for a _____.

I) I may see Aretha Franklin, Garth Brooks, Slayer, Pearl Jam or the local rap, rock or country group when I attend a music _____.

J) They have computers here and assistants to help me find information, where I can read and learn about just about anything.

K) Here, I can lift weights, go for a swim, join an aerobics class, play volleyball and shoot hoops. It is a _____ center.

Home Resources — ACROSS

1) I can easily keep up with current events on a daily basis or get lost in an adventure when I participate in this activity.

2) Indoors or outdoors I can watch my fruits flourish.

3) Model cars, sewing, woodwork, crafts, all make up having a _____.

4) It is best to be alone and in a quiet place for relaxation or _____.

5) Add a little bit of this and a little bit of that. I call this kitchen activity _____.

6) Many times this leisure time activity requires tools and elbow grease _____ maintenance.

7) These friends require much tender loving care and feeding.

8) Lets sit around the table or on the floor and play _____.

9) Sometimes this makes me relax and sometimes I dance, I may even sing.

10) Entertaining others or having your friends over to share a meal or fun is being _____.

11) Too much of this will steal away time from all of the other activities.

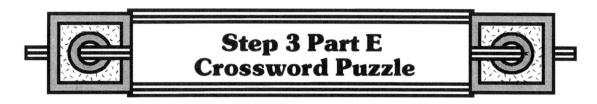

Step 3 Part E
Crossword Puzzle

Name _____   Date _____

Step 3 Part E
Emergency Numbers

Service	Name of Agency	Phone Number
Emergency Services		**Dial 911**
Hospital		
Alcoholics Anonymous		
Mental Health Services		
Suicide Prevention		
Department of Social Services (day number)		
Department of Social Services (night number)		
Chemical Dependency Support Group		
Rape Crisis Center		
Frequently Called Numbers		

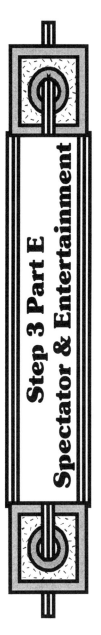

Step 3 Part E
Spectator & Entertainment

Activity	Facility	Address	Phone	Times	How to Get There	Other

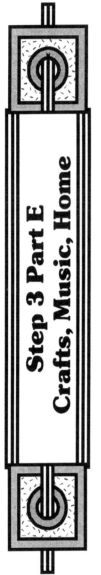

Step 3 Part E
Crafts, Music, Home

Activity	Facility	Address	Phone	Times	How to Get There	Other

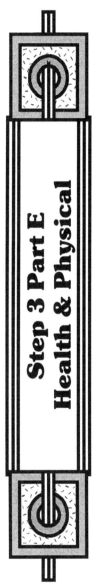

Step 3 Part E
Health & Physical

Activity	Facility	Address	Phone	Times	How to Get There	Other

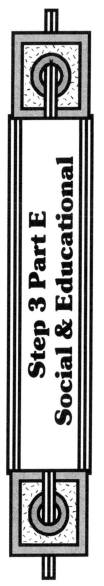

Step 3 Part E
Social & Educational

Activity	Facility	Address	Phone	Times	How to Get There	Other

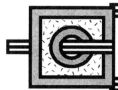

Step 3 Part E
Community Map

The therapist needs to place a map of the participant's local community on this page. It is recommended that the therapist also highlight, number or otherwise note the important leisure and health resource centers on the map for the participant. Use the bottom of this page to type in the names of the resource centers that are highlighted on the map.

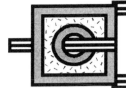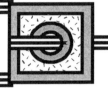

Step 3 Part F
Things I Enjoy

1)   Fill in 5 activities that you enjoy in each area.
2)   Place a check in the category to show who else participates in the activity with you.
3)   Fill in appropriate cost.
4)   Fill in how often you participate in the activity.

A)   Spectator, entertainment

activity	alone	family	friends	cost	how often
1.					
2.					
3.					
4.					
5.					

B)   Arts, crafts, music, drama, dance, home activities

activity	alone	family	friends	cost	how often
1.					
2.					
3.					
4.					
5.					

C)   Exercise, games, sports, physical activities, health

activity	alone	family	friends	cost	how often
1.					
2.					
3.					
4.					
5.					

D)   Educational, cultural, collecting, volunteerism, social activities

activity	alone	family	friends	cost	how often
1.					
2.					
3.					
4.					
5.					

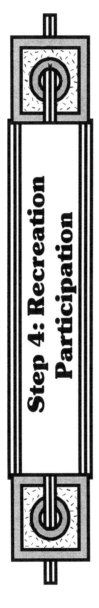

Step 4: Recreation Participation

This step is participatory as opposed to educational. You actively do something. Participate in at least one leisure activity in each of the four leisure levels (1, 2, 3, 4). There is NO participation in the unhealthy, negative levels. To be sure that you understand the meaning of the four positive levels, review the chart of the levels shown in Step 3.

For each activity, write the type of activity, the date and time you did the activity and the amount of time you participated.

Level	Activity	Date	Time	Length	Description of what you did and what you felt
4					
3					
2					
1					

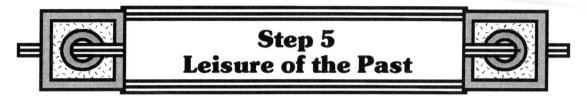

Step 5
Leisure of the Past

Name _____ Date _____

List significant or important leisure activities that you have participated in the past. Put Unhealthy Negative Choices, including Levels Lost Freedom, -1 and -2 on the second page and Healthy Positive Choices including Levels 1, 2, 3, 4 and Cathartic Level on the third page. Answer these questions for each activity:

- What leisure level was I participating on?
- When did I start and stop these activities?
- What was going on in my life at the time?
- Who got me into or out of these activities?

Also answer the questions on the fourth page.
When you are finished, share Step 5 with a counselor or in a group therapy session.

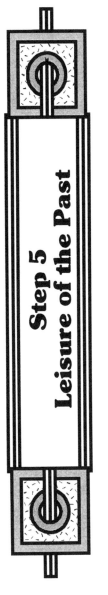

Step 5
Leisure of the Past

Unhealthy Choices

Activity Choice	Level	Start	Stop	What was going on?	Who got me involved?

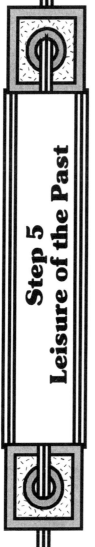

Step 5
Leisure of the Past

Healthy Choices

Activity Choice	Level	Start	Stop	What was going on?	Who got me involved?

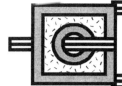 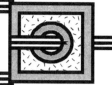

Step 5
Leisure of the Past

My feelings about my past leisure participation are ...

Would I be better off if I changed my lifestyle? Why?

Does anything now prevent me from healthy positive participation?

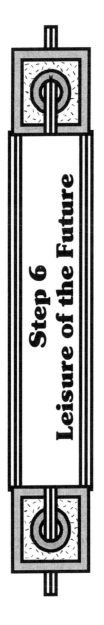

Step 6
Leisure of the Future

Name _____ Date _____

List five Leisure Interests with a specific plan for each. When you are finished, go over these plans with your counselor and note any changes that need to be made.

Activity	Time	Cost	With Whom?	Training	Benefits	Barriers

Is there anything that might prevent these activities from taking place?

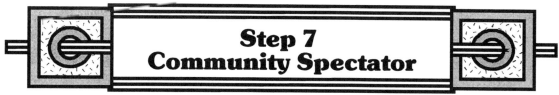

Step 7
Community Spectator

Name _____ Date _____

Participate as a spectator within the community. Write about the experience, share it with a counselor or in group therapy.

What was the activity?

My **thoughts** about the activity ...

My **feelings** about the activity ...

Will I do it again? Why?

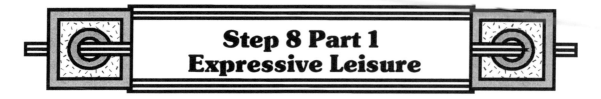

Step 8 Part 1
Expressive Leisure

Name _____ Date _____

Participate in an expressive leisure activity in the areas of arts, crafts, music, drama, dance and home activities. Activity 1 and Activity 2 should be in different areas. Write about the experience. Share it with a counselor or in group therapy.

What was the activity?

My **thoughts** about the activity ...

My **feelings** about the activity ...

Will I do it again? Why?

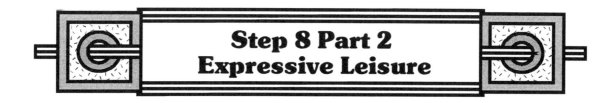

Step 8 Part 2
Expressive Leisure

Name _____   Date _____

Participate in an expressive leisure activity in the areas of arts, crafts, music, drama, dance and home activities. Activity 1 and Activity 2 should be in different areas. Write about the experience. Share it with a counselor or in group therapy.

What was the activity?

My **thoughts** about the activity ...

My **feelings** about the activity ...

Will I do it again? Why?

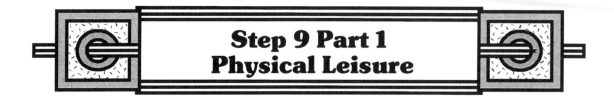

Step 9 Part 1
Physical Leisure

Name _____   Date _____

Participate in a physical leisure activity in the areas of exercise, games, sports, health or physical activities. Activity 1 and Activity 2 should be in different areas. Write about the experience. Share it with a counselor or in group therapy.

What was the activity?

My **thoughts** about the activity ...

My **feelings** about the activity ...

Will I do it again? Why?

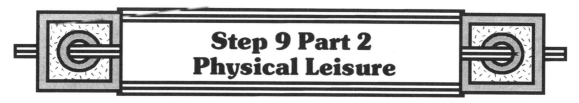

Step 9 Part 2
Physical Leisure

Name _____ Date _____

Participate in a physical leisure activity in the areas of exercise, games, sports, health or physical activities. Activity 1 and Activity 2 should be in different areas. Write about the experience. Share it with a counselor or in group therapy.

What was the activity?

My **thoughts** about the activity ...

My **feelings** about the activity ...

Will I do it again? Why?

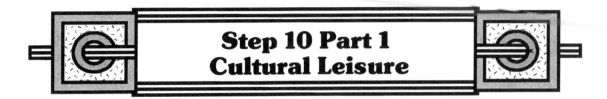

Step 10 Part 1
Cultural Leisure

Name _____ Date _____

Participate in a cultural leisure activity in the areas of education, culture, collecting, volunteering or socializing. Activity 1 and Activity 2 should be in different areas. Write about the experience. Share it with a counselor or in group therapy.

What was the activity?

My **thoughts** about the activity ...

My **feelings** about the activity ...

Will I do it again? Why?

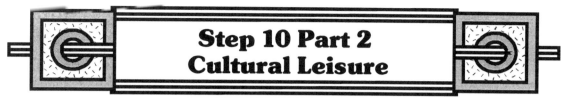

Step 10 Part 2
Cultural Leisure

Name _____ Date _____

Participate in a cultural leisure activity in the areas of education, culture, collecting, volunteering or socializing. Activity 1 and Activity 2 should be in different areas. Write about the experience. Share it with a counselor or in group therapy.

What was the activity?

My **thoughts** about the activity ...

My **feelings** about the activity ...

Will I do it again? Why?

Step 11: Post Discharge Leisure Participation

Name _____   Date _____

Congratulations!!!

You are free and ready to participate in recreation activities of your own choice, time and place!!

I choose to ...

Write about your experiences and share it with family, friends and others!

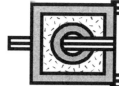 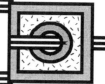

Step 11: Post Discharge Leisure Participation Level

Name _____   Date _____

A. Leisure Activities that I have participated in within the last 30 days	B. Leisure Level		C. Times I participated in the last 30 days		D. Activity Points
		X		=	
		X		=	
		X		=	
		X		=	
		X		=	
		X		=	
		X		=	
		X		=	
		X		=	
		X		=	
		X		=	
		X		=	
		X		=	
		X		=	
		X		=	
		X		=	
		X		=	
		X		=	
Totals for columns C and D					

Level of Participation: Total of Column D / Total of Column C _____

Circle the best answer concerning the use of your leisure time
1. It is excellent and needs no changing.
2. I enjoy my leisure time but it needs minor changes.
3. I am aware of the changes I need to make and feel confident I will make them.
4. I will need some assistance with my leisure participation.
5. I need to review steps of the **Leisure Step Up Workbook** beginning with Step ___.

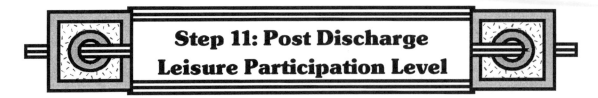

Step 11: Post Discharge Leisure Participation Level

A) Start today and keep track (on a daily basis) of all leisure activities that you participate in for the next 30 days.
B) Give each activity points from the Leisure Level Model.
C) Fill in how many times you participate in each activity.
D) Multiply column B times column C and put the answer in column D.
E) Count up the number of times you participated in activities in column C and put it at the bottom of column C.
F) Add or subtract in column D to get the total and put it at the bottom of column D.
G) Divide the total in column D by the total number of activities in column C to get your average level of participation shown in the chart below.

Leisure Participation Scale

Cathartic Level	Participation in at least one leisure activity with a great deal of emotional release. The event resulted in personal growth.
Level 4	Participation is creative, inventive, imaginative. Be cautious to not spend excessive time in your own world.
Level 2 to 4	Participation seems to be in balance and on a therapeutic level. Leisure pursuits are enjoyable, expressive, active and helpful in solving problems.
Level 1 to 2	Participation spectator. Be cautious that you don't let life pass you by. Also, negative/harmful activity participation can jeopardize the balance in your life.
Level 0	Participation co-dependent. You need to talk, trust, feel, think and live for yourself. Perhaps unhealthy, negative choices are highly influencing your behaviors.
Level -1 to -2	Participation harmful/hurting. These choices may seem fun and harmless but are often driven by anger or unmet needs. Leisure counseling and education can help you attain a higher leisure level or quality of life.
LOST FREEDOM	Counseling may be necessary to restoring you to a healthy, positive level of participation. Seek help, direction and support from a friend, family member, clergy or counselor. Freedom can be restored and it is worth the trouble.

Note: Quality of leisure is not just how many points you scored. Participation at a high level alone does not necessarily mean that you are enjoying yourself. Also you must not get discouraged with a low score. Since you control your own leisure choices, you can change toward healthy positive choices.